# 5-Ingredients Keto Diet Cookbook In 30 Minutes Book 2

By Stephanie Cooper

You agree that by continuing to read this book, where appropriate and/or necessary, you shall consult a professional (including but not limited to your doctor, attorney, or financial advisor or such other advisor as needed) before using any of the suggested remedies, techniques, or information in this book.

Table of Contents

# MOZZARELLA CHICKEN CASSEROLE



## Ingredients

2 lbs chicken breasts, cooked and cubed

1/4 cup pesto

8 oz cream cheese, softened

8 oz mozzarella, cubed

1/4-1/2 cup heavy cream

Nutritional info (per serving): 727 calories; 59.3 g fat; 2.7 g total carbs; 36.1 g protein

## Directions

1. Combine pesto, cream cheese and heavy cream until well mixed.
2. Add chicken and cubed mozzarella to the mixture.
3. Spray a casserole dish with cooking oil and transfer the mixture into it.
4. Heat the oven to 400F. Sprinkle with some shredded mozzarella on top and bake for 25 minutes and serve immediately.

# MUG LASAGNA

Servings: 1

Cook time: 10 minutes

## Ingredients

1/3 zucchini, thinly sliced

6-8 tablespoons full fat ricotta cheese

3 tablespoons shredded full-fat mozzarella

6-8 tablespoons sugar-free marinara

Italian seasoning

Nutritional info (per serving): 371 calories; 23.4 g fat; 7.7 g total carbs; 31.4 g protein

## Directions

1. Take a mug and, add 1 tablespoon of marinara and spread it evenly in the mug.
2. Add a layer of sliced zucchini.
3. Add 1 tablespoon of ricotta on the top.
4. Add more layers of sliced zucchini and ricotta until the mug is full.
5. Heat in microwave for 4-5 minutes at high.
6. After that top it with the Italian seasoning and serve immediately.

# BERRY COBBLER

Servings: 2

Cook time: 6 minutes

## Ingredients

1 cup fresh or frozen berries

1/4 teaspoon coconut flour

3 tablespoons almond flour

3 teaspoons xylitol

1 tablespoon butter, melted

Nutritional info (per serving): **166 calories;** 11.7 g fat; 3.9 g total carbs; 0.6 g protein

## Directions

1. Mix berries, coconut flour and 2 teaspoons xylitol in a mug.
2. Heat in microwave for 2 minutes and take out from the oven.
3. Take a bowl, add almond flour, melted butter, 1 teaspoon xylitol, and mix well.
4. Microwave the topping for 30 seconds, stirring halfway through.
5. Sprinkle this topping on the berry mixture and serve.

# AVOCADO AND BERRY SMOOTHIE

Servings: 2

Cook time: 5 minutes

## Ingredients

1 cup fresh spinach

1⁄2 cup berries, fresh/frozen

1⁄2 avocado

1 cup full-fat coconut milk

1 scoop protein powder

Nutritional info (per serving): 404 calories; 8.5 g fat; 14.9 g total carbs; 14.7 g protein

## Directions

1. Take a blender, add avocado, spinach, berries, coconut milk, protein powder, ice and blend it until frothy.
2. Serve in 2 glasses.

# CHICKEN TENDERS

Servings: 4

Cook time: 15 minutes

## Ingredients

1 package chicken tenders

1 cup almond flour

1 egg, beaten

salt and pepper, to taste

Nutritional info (per serving): **299 calories; 16.3 g fat; 8.5 g total carbs; 8.9 g protein**

## Directions

1. Put chicken tenders into a bowl and season with salt and pepper.
2. Spray the Air Fryer basket with the cooking spray.
3. Put egg and flour into separate bowls.
4. Dip each chicken tender in flour, then dip in egg and coat with flour again.
5. Put chicken tenders into Air Fryer basket and cook at 350F for 10 minutes and serve hot.

# KETO COCKTAIL

Servings: 2

Cook time: 10 minutes

## Ingredients

4 blueberries

2 oz dry gin

1/2 oz lime juice

1 teaspoon powdered erythritol

club soda

Nutritional info (per serving): 139 calories; 0.1 g fat; 2.9 g total carbs; 0.2 g protein

## Directions

1. Put blueberries into a cocktail shaker and shake until they release juice.
2. Add erythritol, gin, lime juice, ice cubes and shake again.
3. Put into glasses, pour club soda on top and serve.

# SHAMROCK SHAKE

Servings: 1

Cook time: 5 minutes

## Ingredients

1/2 medium avocado

1 oz dairy-free vanilla protein powder

1/2 cup Almond Coconut Milk

1/8 teaspoon peppermint extract

1 tablespoon dark chocolate chips

Nutritional info (per serving): 224 calories; 17.9 g fat; 7.8 g total carbs; 3.1 g protein

## Directions

1. In a blender, put avocado, peppermint extract, protein powder, almond coconut milk, ice cubes and blend until frothy and creamy.
2. Top with dark chocolate chips and serve.

# MEXICAN CHICKEN CASSEROLE

Servings: 8

Cook time:
25 minutes

## Ingredients

3 cups shredded
chicken, cooked

16 oz salsa

8 oz cream cheese

8 oz shredded
cheddar cheese

3/4 teaspoon taco
seasoning

Nutritional info (per
serving): 298
calories; 21.1 g fat;
5.5 g total carbs;
22.2 g protein

## Directions

1. Put chicken, 4 oz
   shredded cheese, cream
   cheese, salsa,, 1/2
   teaspoon taco seasoning
   into a bowl and mix
   until combined.
2. Grease a baking tray
   with a cooking spray
   and put chicken on it.
3. Heat the oven to 400F
   and bake for 20 minutes
   or until fully cooked.

# LOW CARB GREEN SMOOTHIE

Servings: 2

Cook time: 7 minutes

## Ingredients

1 cup baby spinach

1/2 cup cilantro

1 inch ginger, peeled

3/4 cucumber, peeled

1 cup frozen avocado

Nutritional info (per serving): 146 calories; 11.3 g fat; 5 g total carbs; 3 g protein

## Directions

1. Combine all ingredients and 1 cup ice cold water in a blender and blend until smooth.
2. Serve immediately or store in a mason jar in refrigerator.

# BROILED CHICKEN WITH GARLIC

Servings: 4

Cook time: 20 minutes

## Ingredients

1 1/2 lbs boneless skinless chicken thighs

1-2 jars artichoke hearts

2 tablespoons minced garlic

2 tablespoons dried oregano

salt and pepper, to taste

Nutritional info (per serving): 281 calories; 16.6 g fat; 5.9 g total carbs; 27.1 g protein

## Directions

1. Put chicken breasts and artichoke hearts into a bowl, mix well and let it marinate for 20 minutes.
2. Add oregano, minced garlic and season with salt and pepper.
3. Broil for 18-25 minutes on high heat.
4. Serve when chicken is cooked and crisped.

# ROSEMARY CHICKEN KABOBS



## Ingredients

3 boneless-skinless chicken breasts

8 bamboo skewers

3 garlic cloves, minced

1/4 cup olive oil

2 tablespoons chopped rosemary

Nutritional info (per serving): **395 calories; 21.7 g fat; 12.8 g total carbs; 38.2 g protein**

## Directions

1. Cut chicken breasts in bite-size pieces and soak bamboo skewers in water for 15 minutes.
2. Combine all ingredients in a large bowl and mix well to coat the chicken properly.
3. Now thread chicken chunks on the bamboo skewers.
4. Heat the grill to 375F and grill chicken for 12-15 minutes flipping every 3 minutes.

# BACON WRAPPED SCALLOPS

Servings: 4

Cook time: 25 minutes

## Ingredients

16 sea scallops

8 slices bacon, cut in half crosswise

olive oil for drizzling

16 toothpicks

salt and pepper, to taste

Nutritional info (per serving): 532 calories; 10.5 g fat; 8 g total carbs; 23 g protein

## Directions

1. Wrap one scallop in bacon slice and secure with the help of a toothpick.
2. Repeat the process for other scallops.
3. Put all scallops on the baking tray, season with salt and pepper, and drizzle some olive oil on the top.
4. Heat the oven to 425F and cook in the oven for 12-15 minutes.
5. Remove from the oven and serve immediately.

# QUICK CAULIFLOWER MAC & CHEESE

Servings: 1

Cook time: 7 minutes

## Ingredients

3/4 cup frozen cauliflower florets

1 oz shredded cheddar cheese

1 tablespoon heavy cream

Nutritional info (per serving): 183 calories; 14.4 g fat; 3.3 g total carbs; 8.5 g protein

## Directions

1. Put cauliflower florets into a microwave safe bowl, cover and microwave for 1 minute.
2. Chop cauliflower and put into the microwave for another minute.
3. Remove from the microwave, add shredded cheese and microwave for 10 more seconds.
4. Add heavy cream and stir properly before serving.

# ROASTED CHICKEN THIGHS

Servings: 8

Cook time: 20 minutes

## Ingredients

2 lbs boneless chicken thighs

1 tablespoon chili powder

1 tablespoon olive oil

fresh cilantro, for garnish

salt and pepper, to taste

Nutritional info (per serving): 188 calories; 12.8 g fat; 0.6 g total carbs; 17.2 g protein

## Directions

1. Line a large baking tray with parchment paper and put chicken on it.
2. Drizzle with some olive oil and season with salt, pepper and chili powder.
3. Heat the oven to 375F and roast in the oven for 15 minutes or until cooked.
4. Garnish with fresh cilantro and serve hot.

# BUNLESS BURGER



## Ingredients

1 lb ground beef

1 tablespoon Montreal Steak Seasoning

1 tablespoon Worcestershire sauce

salt and pepper, to taste

olive oil (optional)

Nutritional info (per serving): 403 calories; 24.6 g fat; 1.1 g total carbs; 39.5 g protein

## Directions

1. Mix beef, Worcestershire sauce steak seasoning and olive oil in a bowl.
2. Shape the mixture into 3 burger sized patties.
3. Top the patties with salt and pepper
4. Heat the grill, oil a grater and grill until cooked.
5. You can serve it with caramelized onions.

# CHICKEN SALAD

Servings: 2

Cook time: 10 minutes

## Ingredients

10 oz boneless chicken breasts

6 thin-cut slices bacon

1 large avocado, sliced

4 cups mixed leafy greens

4 tablespoons Keto Ranch Dressing

Nutritional info (per serving): 484 calories; 29.7 g fat; 7.7 g total carbs; 43.5 g protein

## Directions

1. Season chicken breasts with salt and pepper.
2. Heat a large pan until hot, grease it with ghee.
3. Add chicken breast and cook for 5-6 minutes until golden and crispy.
4. Heat the oven to 400F, remove from the pan and put it into the oven for 10 minutes until cooked.
5. Remove from the oven and slice into small pieces.
6. Combine sliced chicken, leafy greens and sliced avocado in a bowl.
7. Top with Ranch Dressing and serve.

# TURMERIC LATTE



## Ingredients

16 oz warmed almond milk

2 teaspoons turmeric powder

1 packet of Keto Instant Coffee

1/2 teaspoon ground cinnamon

1 teaspoon vanilla extract

Nutritional info (per serving): 54 calories; 3.2 g fat; 4.1 g total carbs; 1.2 g protein

## Directions

1. Combine all ingredients in a blender and blend until frothy and creamy.
2. Pour into 2 glasses and serve.

# INSTANT POT CRACK CHICKEN

Servings: 4

Cook time: 30 minutes

## Ingredients

2 lbs chicken breasts

12 oz cream cheese, cubed

1/2 cup Cheddar cheese

8 oz bacon, crumbled

1 oz packet Dry Ranch Seasoning

Nutritional info (per serving): 945 calories; 35.7 g fat; 4.5 g total carbs; 80.6 g protein

## Directions

1. Pour 1 cup water into the inner pot.
2. Add chicken, cubed cream cheese and seasonings.
3. Set the cooker on high and cook for 12 minutes.
4. Take out the chicken and shred it with a fork.
5. Put the chicken back into the pot and add cheddar cheese and bacon crumbles into the pot.
6. Mix well and close the cooker for 5 minutes to melt cheese (without turning the heat on) before serving.

# GRILLED LIME SHRIMP

Servings: 2

Cook time: 10 minutes

## Ingredients

1 1/2 oz smoked turkey breast, sliced

1 1/2 oz cream cheese

1 teaspoon Sriracha sauce

1 large iceberg lettuce leaf

5 toothpicks

Nutritional info (per serving): 97 calories; 7.4 g fat; 2.1 g total carbs; 5.6 g protein

## Directions

1. Put the lettuce leaf on a plate.
2. Add layers of turkey, sriracha and cream cheese on it.
3. Roll the lettuce leaf carefully and secure it with the help of toothpicks.
4. Slice into 5 roll ups and serve.

# EGG WRAPS

Servings: 2

Cook time: 5 minutes

## Ingredients

4 eggs

1 avocado, thinly sliced

butter

salt and pepper, to taste

Nutritional info (per serving): 305 calories; 24.8 g fat; 9.4 g total carbs; 14.6 g protein

## Directions

1. Heat a pan over a medium heat and add some butter.
2. Put egg into a bowl and whisk it well with a fork.
3. Pour the egg into the pan and sprinkle with seasoning on top.
4. Cook for 30 second and flip on the other side with a spatula.
5. Put it on a plate, top with avocado filling and roll up.
6. Repeat for all the eggs.

# ZUCCHINI CHIPS

Servings: 4

Cook time: 30 minutes

## Ingredients

2 large zucchini, thinly sliced

1 1/2 cup freshly grated Parmesan cheese

marinara sauce, for dipping

salt and pepper, to taste

Nutritional info (per serving): 187 calories; 11 g fat; 7 g total carbs; 16.4 g protein

## Directions

1. Put zucchini slices into a bowl and season with salt and pepper.
2. Put slices on a baking tray and top each slice with Parmesan cheese.
3. Heat oven to 400F and bake in the oven for 20 minutes.
4. Serve with Marinara sauce.

# CAULIFLOWER HUMMUS

Servings: 6

Cook time: 25 minutes

## Ingredients

1 medium cauliflower, cut into florets

1/3 cup tahini

1 clove garlic, peeled

1/3 cup olive oil

3 tablespoons lemon juice

Nutritional info (per serving): 190 calories; 19.2 g fat; 3.9 g total carbs; 2.4 g protein

## Directions

1. Put cauliflower florets into a bowl, drizzle olive oil on top and season with salt.
2. Preheat the oven to 425F and bake in the oven for 20 minutes or until tender.
3. Remove from the oven and set aside to cool.
4. Combine all the ingredients and roasted cauliflower in a food processor and process until creamy.
5. Add water to get desired consistency.

# TAHINI VINAIGRETTE



## Ingredients

1/2 cup Tahini

1 garlic clove, minced

1 tablespoon Sriracha

4 tablespoons lemon juice

salt and pepper, to taste

Nutritional info (per serving): 372 calories; 32.5 g fat; 6.9 g total carbs; 10.2 g protein

## Directions

1. Combine all the ingredients, 3/4 cup water and season with salt and black pepper.
2. Wisk all the ingredients together and serve.

# PARMESAN TOMATOES

Servings: 6

Cook time: 25 minutes

## Ingredients

6 small tomatoes, halved

1/2 cup grated Parmesan cheese

1 tablespoon olive oil

salt and black pepper, to taste

Nutritional info (per serving): 72 calories; 4.8 g fat; 3.8 g total carbs; 4 g protein

## Directions

1. Season halved tomatoes with salt and pepper and drizzle some olive oil on top.
2. Put tomatoes on a baking tray and add Parmesan cheese.
3. Heat the oven to 400F and roast in the oven for 15-20 minutes.
4. Remove from the oven when cheese is melted and serve hot.

# CREAM CHEESE DIP

Servings: 10

Cook time: 10 minutes

## Ingredients

8 oz full-fat cream cheese

1 cup shredded Cheddar cheese

1/2 cup chopped pimento-stuffed olives

1/2 cup mayonnaise

1 garlic clove, crushed

Nutritional info (per serving): 202 calories; 12.6 g fat; 1.9 g total carbs; 6.2 g protein

## Directions

1. Whisk together all the ingredients with an electric mixer until well combined.
2. Put into the freezer for 2-3 hours.
3. Serve in a serving dish.

# CAPRESE ZOODLES

Servings: 4

Cook time: 25 minutes

## Ingredients

4 large zucchinis, made into zoodles

2 cups cherry tomatoes, halved

1/4 cup fresh basil leaves

1 cup mozzarella balls, quartered

2 tablespoons extra-virgin olive oil

2 tablespoons balsamic vinegar

Nutritional info (per serving): 243 calories; 15.4 g fat; 6.5 g total carbs; 12.7 g protein

## Directions

1. Put zucchini noodles into a bowl, season with salt and pepper and drizzle some olive oil the top.
2. Add mozzarella, tomatoes, basil and toss to combine well.
3. Drizzle balsamic vinegar on top and serve.

# CAULIFLOWER TOAST WITH AVOCADO

Servings: 2

Cook time: 20 minutes

## Ingredients

1 head cauliflower, grated

1 medium avocado, chopped

1/2 cup Mozzarella cheese

1 egg

1/2 teaspoon garlic powder

Nutritional info (per serving): 312 calories; 19.7 g fat; 12.8 g total carbs; 17.3 g protein

## Directions

1. Put grated cauliflower into a bowl and heat in a microwave for 8 minutes.
2. Add mozzarella cheese, egg,, garlic powder and mix until well combined.
3. Season with salt and pepper
4. Put it on a baking tray in the form of even little squares.
5. Heat oven to 425F, put it into the oven and bake for 18 minutes.
6. Put avocado, salt, pepper into a bowl and mesh avocado until smooth.
7. Transfer the cauliflower toast to a serving tray, add mashed avocado on top and serve.

# CHOCOLATE CHIP WAFFLES

Servings: 2

Cook time: 15 minutes

## Ingredients

2 scoops keto protein powder

2 eggs

2 tablespoon butter, melted

1 2/3 oz sugar-free chocolate chips

2 tablespoons monkfruit liquid

Nutritional info (per serving): 409 calories; 18.3 g fat; 9.2 g total carbs; 28.5 g protein

## Directions

1. Combine 2 scoops of protein powder, melted butter and egg yolks in a bowl.
2. Whisk egg whites in another bowl.
3. Combine the two mixture, add chocolate chips and a pinch of salt.
4. Heat the waffle maker, pour the mixture onto the waffle maker and cook until done.
5. Drizzle some maple syrup on top and serve.

# CHICKEN TOMATO BITES

Servings: 6

Cook time: 15 minutes

## Ingredients

12 Campari cocktail sized tomatoes

2/3 cup chopped cooked chicken

1/3 cup pesto sauce

1 1/2 tablespoons mayonnaise

⅓ cup grated Mozzarella cheese

Nutritional info (per serving): 215 calories; 14.1 g fat; 9.7 g total carbs; 12.6 g protein

## Directions

1. Cut off top of tomatoes and scoop out all the insides.
2. Keep the tomatoes shells aside.
3. Heat a pan on a medium heat until hot.
4. Add chicken, pesto sauce to the pan. Stir and cook for 5-6 minutes.
5. Add mayonnaise and remove from the stove.
6. Fill tomatoes shells with the mixture and top with cheese before serving.

# CHOCOLATE LAVA CAKE

Servings: 2

Cook time: 16 minutes

## Ingredients

2 oz dark chocolate

1 tablespoon almond flour

2 oz butter

2 eggs

2 tablespoons powdered sweetener

Nutritional info (per serving): 439 calories; 40 g fat; 7 g total carbs; 8.5 g protein

## Directions

1. Beat the eggs in a bowl.
2. Melt butter and chocolate.
3. Add the egg mixture, almond flour and sweetener and mix until you get a dough-like consistency.
4. Heat the oven to 350F, pour the mixture into 2 pre-greased ramekins and bake in the oven for 9 minutes.
5. Put on a plate, dust some powdered sweetener on top and serve.

# GUACAMOLE

Servings: 6

Cook time: 15 minutes

## Ingredients

3 avocados, mashed

1/2 large onion, diced

1/2 cup tomato, diced

1/2 lime, juiced

salt and pepper, to taste

Nutritional info (per serving): 170 calories; 14.8 g fat; 9 g total carbs; 2.3 g protein

## Directions

1. Combine mashed avocado, lime juice, onion and tomato in a bowl and stir well.
2. Season with salt and pepper to taste and serve.

# CAULIFLOWER CHEESE BITES

Servings: 2

Cook time: 20 minutes

## Ingredients

5 egg whites

1/2 cup cauliflower, riced

1 cup cheese, shredded

butter

Nutritional info (per serving): 108 calories; 4.4 g fat; 2.2 g total carbs; 14.4 g protein

## Directions

1. Combine riced cauliflower, shredded cheese and egg whites in a bowl and mix well.
2. Grease muffin tin with butter and put 1 tablespoon of the mixture to the bottom of the muffin tin.
3. Add some shredded cheese on top.
4. Heat the oven to 400F and bake in the oven for 15 minutes.
5. Remove from the oven and serve immediately.

# CHOCOLATE FAT BOMBS

Servings: 4

Cook time: 30 minutes

## Ingredients

3/4 cup cocoa powder

3/4 cup coconut oil, melted

3 drops liquid sweetener

1 teaspoon vanilla extract

Nutritional info (per serving): **391** calories; 43 g fat; 8.8 g total carbs; 3.3 g protein

## Directions

1. Mix cocoa powder and coconut oil in a bowl until smooth.
2. Add vanilla extract, sweetener and stir well.
3. Pour the mixture into the molt.
4. Freeze for 25 minutes and enjoy.

# CRUNCHY NO BAKE COOKIE

Servings: 20

Cook time: 30 minutes

## Ingredients

1 1/3 cups creamy peanut butter

2 cups coconut flakes

2 tablespoons cocoa powder

2 tablespoons butter, melted

2 teaspoons vanilla extract

Nutritional info (per serving): 135 calories; 11.6 g fat; 5.9 g total carbs; 4 g protein

## Directions

1. Combine all the ingredients in a bowl and mix until well combined.
2. Line a large baking tray with parchment paper.
3. Scoop batter onto the tray and slightly press with a spoon to make it in a cookie shape.
4. Put the tray into the freezer for 30 minutes.
5. Store cookies in an airtight container in a freezer.

# SAUSAGE KALE SOUP

Servings: 6

Cook time: 25 minutes

## Ingredients

1 lb Italian turkey sausage, sliced

8 oz chopped kale

15 oz diced tomatoes

1/2 cup diced onion

4 cups chicken broth

Nutritional info (per serving): 182 calories; 8.4 g fat; 9.4 g total carbs; 15.8 g protein

## Directions

1. Put turkey sausages into your instant pot and set to Saute mode.
2. Add tomatoes, onions and chicken broth to the pot.
3. Close the lid, set to Manual mode and cook on High for 15 minutes.
4. When cooker turns off, let it sit for 10 minutes and then release the steam from the cooker.
5. Put chopped kale and 1/2 a cup of water into a microwave safe bowl and heat in the oven for 3 minutes.
6. Drain water and set aside kale
7. Open the lid and add kale before serving.

# SMOKED SALMON CEVICHE

Servings: 1

Cook time: 10 minutes

## Ingredients

1/4 cucumber, cut into thin sticks

2.8 oz smoked salmon, sliced

1/2 large avocado, sliced

1/2 lime

cilantro, to garnish

Nutritional info (per serving): 322 calories; 14.8 g fat; 8.2 g total carbs; 21.2 g protein

## Directions

1. Combine cucumbers, smoked salmon, avocado in a serving plate.
2. Squeeze half a lemon on top.
3. Season with black pepper, garnish with cilantro on top and serve.

# SMOKED SALMON CEVICHE M

Servings: 6

Cook time: 8 minutes

## Ingredients

2 avocados, pitted

1 1/2 cups coconut milk

1/4 cup erythritol sweetener

2 tablespoons lime juice

Nutritional info (per serving): 246 calories; 24.1 g fat; 9.5 g total carbs; 2.7 g protein

## Directions

1. Combine all the ingredients in a high speed blender and blend until smooth and creamy.
2. Pour the liquid into 6 popsicle molds and put popsicle sticks into the center of the molds.
3. Put into the freezer until completely solidified before serving.

# COCONUT NUTELLA

Servings: 16

Cook time: 10 minutes

## Ingredients

2 cups raw hazelnuts

6 tablespoons raw cacao powder

2 tablespoons coconut oil

1/2 cup full fat coconut milk, canned

1 teaspoon vanilla extract

Nutritional info (per serving): 70 calories; 2.2 g fat; 2.6 g total carbs; 1.7 g protein

## Directions

1. Preheat the oven to 325 °F
2. Roast hazelnuts in the oven for 10 minutes.
3. Rub off the skin by using a paper towel.
4. Add roasted hazelnuts, cacao powder, coconut oil, coconut milk, vanilla extract and stevia (if desired) in blender and blend into Nutella consistency.

# TIRAMISU MOUSSE



## Ingredients

1/2 cup mascarpone cheese

1 teaspoon baking cocoa powder

1 tablespoon erythritol

Nutritional info (per serving): 194 calories; 10.5 g fat; 1.4 g total carbs; 9.9 g protein

## Directions

1. Combine all ingredients in a bowl and whisk until it becomes smooth and creamy.
2. Serve immediately or store in a refrigerator up to a day.

# KETO GRANOLA

Servings: 4

Cook time: 25 minutes

## Ingredients

5 tablespoons flaxseed meal

5 tablespoons coconut flakes

1 tablespoon Chia seeds

1 1/2 oz nuts

4 tablespoons liquid sweetener

Nutritional info (per serving): 185 calories; 10.1 g fat; 11 g total carbs; 4.2 g protein

## Directions

1. Combine all ingredients in a bowl and spread evenly on a baking tray.
2. Preheat the oven to 350F and bake in the oven for 20 minutes.
3. Remove from the oven, let it cool and store in an airtight container.

# MINI-SKILLET PIZZA MARGARITA

Servings: 3

Cook time: 20 minutes

## Ingredients

4 egg whites

3 whole eggs

1/2 cup coconut flour

3 tablespoons spaghetti sauce

1/2 cup mozzarella cheese

Nutritional info (per serving): 286 calories; 13.1 g fat; 9.5 g total carbs; 21 g protein

## Directions

1. Wisk 2 egg whites and 3 whole eggs.
2. Add coconut flour, baking powder and whisk until smooth.
3. Heat a greased pan on a low heat, pour the mixture and cook on low heat for 5 minutes.
4. Carefully flip the side and cook for 2 more minutes.
5. Add cheese and spaghetti sauce on top.
6. Broil on low heat until cheese is melted.

# PINEAPPLE CUCUMBER STICKS

Servings: 15

Cook time: 10 minutes

## Ingredients

5 sticks pineapple

5 sticks cucumber

5 sticks jicama

2 lime wedges

1 teaspoon chili lime seasoning

Nutritional info (per serving): 15 calories; 1 g fat; 4 g total carbs; 0 g protein

## Directions

1. Combine cucumber, jicama, pineapple, chili lime seasoning, and lemon juice in a bowl.
2. Toss to coat with the seasoning before serving.

# SALMON ALFREDO

Servings: 3

Cook time: 18 minutes

## Ingredients

3/4 lb salmon

4 medium zucchinis, spiralized

1/5 cup shredded parmesan

8 oz whipping cream

fresh dill to taste

Nutritional info (per serving): 535 calories; 37.1 g fat; 7.1 g total carbs; 34.4 g protein

## Directions

1. Heat the oven to 400F. Season salmon with salt and pepper and bake it for 10 minutes.
2. Remove from the oven and mesh with a fork.
3. Season spiralized zucchini noodles with salt and set aside for 10 minutes.
4. Heat a non stick pan on a medium heat, pour cream into the pan and simmer.
5. Add Parmesan and pepper in the pan and cook on low heat until sauce thickens.
6. Turn off the heat, add zucchini noodles and mix well.
7. Add fresh dill and some shredded Parmesan on top, season to taste and serve.

# ALMOND CRACKERS



## Ingredients

1 cup almond flour

1 tablespoon ground flaxseeds

3 tablespoons water

1/4 teaspoon salt

Nutritional info (per serving): 240 calories; 20 g fat; 6.7 g total carbs; 1 g protein

## Directions

1. Combine all ingredients in a bowl, mix until it takes form of a dough, and set aside for 10 minutes.
2. Put the dough on a non-stick parchment paper and cover it with another parchment paper on the top.
3. Roll the dough to a 3 mm thickness.
4. Remove the parchment paper and cut into rectangles shape.
5. Heat oven to 370F, put crackers on a baking tray and bake in the oven for 20 minutes.
6. Store in an airtight container.

# ALMOND CRACKERS



## Ingredients

3/4 cup almond flour

3 oz strawberries

2 tablespoons granulated Stevia

4 tablespoons cream cheese

1 teaspoon lemon juice

Nutritional info (per serving): 64 calories; 5.4 g fat; 2 g total carbs; 0.3 g protein

## Directions

1. Put strawberries and stevia in a saucepan and cook for 15 minutes on a low heat until a thick syrup forms, stirring occasionally.
2. Combine strawberry sauce, cream cheese, almond flour, lemon juice in a large mixing bowl and beat with an electric mixer on a medium speed.
3. Put the dough into a freezer until hard enough to make balls.
4. Roll into small balls and freeze for 30 minutes.
5. Store in an airtight container up to a month.

# PEPPERONI PIZZA BITES

Servings: 24

Cook time: 18 minutes

## Ingredients

24 slices pepperoni

24 mini mozzarella balls

24 small basil leaves

1 small jar pizza sauce

Nutritional info (per serving): 75 calories; 5.6 g fat; 0.2 g total carbs; 4.9 g protein

## Directions

1. Snip 1/2 inch cut around the edges of pepperoni slices with a shears, in a way that each pepperoni looks like a circular cross.
2. Heat the oven to 400F, put pepperoni in the bottom of a mini muffin pan and bake for 15 minutes.
3. Remove from the oven and put a basil leaf into the bottom of each cup.
4. Add 1/2 teaspoon of pizza sauce, a mini mozzarella ball, and an olive slice on top.
5. Bake in the oven for 3 more minutes until cheese melts and then serve.

# AVOCADO DEVILED EGGS

Servings: 4

Cook time: 10 minutes

## Ingredients

10 eggs, hardboiled

1 ripe avocado

1 lemon, juiced

smoked paprika

1 tablespoon Dijon mustard

Nutritional info (per serving): **196 calories; 7.8 g fat; 7.4 g total carbs; 11.3 g protein**

## Directions

1. Slice eggs in half and remove yolks.
2. Add avocado, egg yolks, lemon juice and mustard in a bowl.
3. Season with salt and pepper.
4. Process in a food processor until smooth.
5. Add the mixture into a piping bag and fill the halved egg whites with this filling.
6. Sprinkle some black pepper and paprika on top and serve.

# BBQ JALAPENO POPPERS

Servings: 12

Cook time: 30 minutes

## Ingredients

6 oz cream cheese

3/4 cup shredded pepper jack cheese

6 slices bacon

6 large jalapenos, halved

2 teaspoons BBQ seasoning

Nutritional info (per serving): 92 calories; 7.9 g fat; 1.8 g total carbs; 3.5 g protein

## Directions

1. Put cream cheese in a microwave safe bowl and microwave for 30-45 seconds.
2. Add half cup pepper jack cheese and BBQ seasoning to the bowl and mix until well combined.
3. Fill jalapenos halves with the cream cheese mixture.
4. Top filled jalapenos with the remaining shredded pepper jack cheese.
5. Now wrap half slice of bacon around each jalapeno.
6. Preheat the oven to 400F, place on a baking tray and cook for 20 minutes and broil for 5 minutes.

# PEPPERMINT HEMP FAT FUDGE

Servings: 13

Cook time: 30 minutes

## Ingredients

3/4 cup coconut oil, melted

1.2 cup dark chocolate chips, melted

1/3 cup Hemp Hearts, soaked

1/2 teaspoon vanilla extract

1 teaspoon peppermint extract

Nutritional info (per serving): 188 calories; 18.2 g fat; 8.9 g total carbs; 1.2 g protein

## Directions

1. Combine all ingredients in a blender and blend well until smooth.
2. Pour mixture into a silicone mold with rectangular cavities.
3. Put in the fridge for 20 minutes.
4. Put fudge on a plate and serve.

# PARMESAN CHEESE CRISPS

Servings: 12

Cook time: 30 minutes

## Ingredients

1 cup shredded Parmesan cheese

1 teaspoon dried basil

Nutritional info (per serving): 36 calories; 2.4 g fat; 0.4 g total carbs; 3.2 g protein

## Directions

1. Spoon Parmesan Cheese on the baking tray in form of small piles.
2. Press with a spoon or hand to evenly flatten.
3. Sprinkle dried basil on top.
4. Heat the oven to 350F and bake for 5 minutes.